MW01247668

TRAUMA STILL
Speaks

WITH WORKBOOK

Part 1

STEVEN O. ALLEN

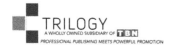

Trauma Still Speaks - Part 1

Trilogy Christian Publishers

A Wholly Owned Subsidary of Trinity Broadcasting Network

2442 Michelle Drive, Tustin, CA 92780

Copyright © 2024 by Steven O. Allen

All Scripture quotations, unless otherwise noted, taken from the New King James Version®. Copyright © 1982 by Thomas Nelson. Used by permission. All rights reserved.

Scripture quotations marked (KJV) taken from The Holy Bible, King James Version. Cambridge Edition: 1769.

All rights reserved, including the right to reproduce this book or portions thereof in any form whatsoever.

For information, address Trilogy Christian Publishing

Rights Department, 2442 Michelle Drive, Tustin, CA 92780.

Trilogy Christian Publishing/ TBN and colophon are trademarks of Trinity Broadcasting Network.

For information about special discounts for bulk purchases, please contact Trilogy Christian Publishing.

Trilogy Disclaimer: The views and content expressed in this book are those of the author and may not necessarily reflect the views and doctrine of Trilogy Christian Publishing or the Trinity Broadcasting Network.

10 9 8 7 6 5 4 3 2 1

Library of Congress Cataloging-in-Publication Data is available.

ISBN 979-8-89333-382-4

ISBN 979-8-89333-383-1

ACKNOWLEDGEMENTS

I would like to take a moment to give thanks to the Lord for allowing me the grace and opportunity to learn, to share what I have learned in this book, and to live the results. I would also like to give thanks to those who have loved and supported me throughout my journey to healing. Christ In Action Ministries (CIAM) partners, Dominion LYFE Institute partners, my closest family and friends, and my prayer partners (you know who you are) that have kept me covered in prayer throughout the process of writing this book. It has taken me quite a while to complete, but it's finally done. May God's blessings multiply in your life.

Contents

INTRODUCTION

Today is Friday July 1, 2022, and I am on a beautifully breathtaking, white sand Caribbean beach with multicolored waters as I begin to write. I am actually watching sailboats and ships of varying sizes, designs, and *purposes* floating in the waves. As I begin to pay closer attention, I observe that a few of these boats are the same ones I had seen the day before, in almost the exact same positions. What I realize is that they are all *immobilized,* or *bound* by their anchors. On the surface, all the right elements that normally create movement and momentum through the waves and the winds are at work.

But there's another object or force at work deep below what is actually visible that stops all forward momentum. Something so small in comparison to the boat itself can halt its movements, stagnate, stall, and stifle all its progression. At best it will *swing on the hook* immobilized as the wind and waves can cause it to drift in a small circle around the chain that's connecting it to the anchor. This is such a powerful concept, because most of us have actually been bound, immobilized, suspended, or anchored by something from the past or present that we may not even be cognizant of.

Today is Tuesday, July 5, 2022. I am grateful to have had the privilege of spending several days on an amazingly beautiful Caribbean Island. Due to sensitivity and my empathy for the peoples' plight, I will not name the particular island. This land has awe-inspiring beauty all along its coastlines, with more beaches than there is time to visit. These bays and the beaches are so gloriously magnetic they attract tourists from all around the world from thousands of miles away. This is a land where nature produces many types of tropical fruits, herbs, and an endless supply of sun, sand, and sea breezes unrivaled by anything that mankind could ever replicate.

I am now cruising at an altitude of 36,000 feet as I pen this, reminiscing about my experiences on this paradise island. During my stay, each morning I was greeted with a sea-swept breeze that felt as if it was straight from heaven as the sun kissed my skin ever so gently. Remarkably, the sand and waves just soothed my feet, as well as my soul, as if it all waited impatiently all night just to touch me. It is a momentary space of bliss and suspended animation where no yesterday or tomorrow even exists, but only *now*. It's a space where *there* doesn't even exist...only *here*. It is a space where only gravity itself can hold you...but barely.

Yet, amongst all this other-worldly beauty, heavenly splendor, and glorious magnificence, you can take just a very short drive to the interior (inner) of the island in any direction, and it's like stepping into a different world altogether. It's a country of two nations and stark contradictions. It's a place where the people are very gracious and generous, but many are forced to live in major oppression and stark poverty, with all the challenges that this brings en masse. But wait a minute; how in the world can this be? To the very unsuspecting outsider, this oasis in the sea seems to be a perfect paradise filled with nothing but majesty and awe. But upon further inspection, you see another truth at work deep behind the scenes—the other side of paradise. On the outer (outward) perimeter is paradise, but deeper in the interior there's peril. Seem familiar?

In this book, we will look in depth into some of the various and common aspects of emotional wounds, damaged emotions, and soul trauma that lurk beneath the surface in an unseen realm of reality.

Furthermore, the terms damaged emotions, wounded emotions, wounded soul, and soul trauma will be used interchangeably. We will not only discuss the problems, signs, and symptoms associated with the effects of damaged emotions, but we will also discuss how to identify the root causes or sources, and the solutions to redemption, renewal, and restoration into a life of inner-healing and emotional wholeness with the freedom that only truth healing can produce.

The subject of inner/emotional healing has gained a lot of attention in the last several years. So many people are living their normal daily lives in need of this healing but are completely unaware they are in need of it. Others are aware that it is needed but are not sure of how or where to get it. In this book, we will discuss ways you can recognize if you need it, as well as some very practical tools to help you begin your process to healing, restoration, freedom, and a new lease on life, despite the traumas you have experienced during your life. Yesterday may have been a traumatic past, but through prayer and process, this book will usher you into a triumphant future.

NOTE:

As a note, any scriptures referenced in this book will be taken from the KJV or NKJV unless otherwise stated.

Chapter 1

---·---

TRAUMATIZATION AND SIGNS
THAT EMOTIONAL HEALING IS NEEDED

Let me begin by making these two statements:

(1) You will never conquer what you will not confront. (2) You will always have what you've always had if you always do what you've always done. These two statements are especially true when there is emotional trauma from the past embedded in your life and etched deeply into your soul's foundation. At best you will only learn how to just manage or suppress the effects of this trauma, even though it will still always find ways to leak out and "speak" when it has been triggered or activated.

The following are some signs that you (or someone you know) may need some emotional healing. This is not at all-inclusive or an exhaustive list, but it will be enough to get us started. You will get more out of this book if you really take time to pray, self-reflect, and meditate through the chapters and do whatever work is recommended in the workbook section. This book is not designed to just be another entertaining book to read, but to engage you, the reader, and to activate you into actions that will foster positive, life-changing results. The good news is that no matter who you are, what hurts or disappointments you have sustained, how badly you were mistreated, misunderstood, misjudged, or how you may have misbehaved, it's not over for you, and you can have a new lease on life.

Psalms 147:3 states, "He heals the brokenhearted and binds up their wounds." As far as I am concerned, the Word of God is the final authority over your circumstances or any situation you could be faced with.

Physical trauma is easily recognizable because it is *outward* and very noticeable. Take a car that's been damaged in an accident, for example. The car can have the doors, windows, bumpers, and fenders all replaced with new ones, and that car may not show any evidence of ever being damaged. Once repaired, it can look perfectly normal from a distance or to an untrained eye. A well-trained professional can inspect this same car and can tell right away if the replaced components are the original ones that came from the factory. They can also discern if the structure beneath the replaced components and what is visible has any damage.

This same thing is true regarding a person who has a physical injury. It is easily recognizable to the person and to others. The person may look, sound, and seem perfectly normal and live a perfectly normal life when the physical injury heals. Often there is little to no evidence that the injury was ever even there, with the exception of maybe a scar.

But what about when the injury or damage is internal? What about when the scars are deep, unhealed emotional wounds that are masked by outward appearances and behaviors? What about when these emotional wounds have festered for months, years, even decades? In many cases, these wounds even last a lifetime, as they go suppressed, masked, and even denied of their very existence. I suggest and truly believe that intense or repeated emotional traumas create emotional wounds and damage to people's souls that can last a lifetime if they go unhealed. I submit to you that the longer the emotional wounds have been there, the more difficult they are to accept in some instances because the person believes that "this is just me," and they have adopted a new normal. In fact, it is very likely that these emotional wounds have even changed the person's personality to some degree, depending upon how deep these wounds are.

Your soul, in its simplest definition, consists of your mind, your will, and your emotions. This is what makes you uniquely who you are as a human, including your personality and character. If the mind, the will, or the emotions get damaged through the wounds of mistreatment, abuse (of any type), neglect, abandonment, or rejection, then the very essence of who you are suffers a negative impact. These unhealed, damaged emotions often sabotage a person's potential, relationships, character, and their life's purpose more often than not. If a person's emotions are damaged from past traumas, certain areas of that person's life will experience some level of stagnation or dysfunction. Unavoidably, they remain stuck in that place until they receive the healing they need, and the residual effects of the wounds are no longer present. Until then, the trauma still speaks.

This is especially true in various types of relationships, even in a person's relationship with themselves. Have you ever heard the phrase "hurt people hurt people"? Well, this is an unfortunate and ugly truth, mainly because you hurt others with the hurt you're hurting with. When there are suppressed or unhealed damaged emotions lurking, you can become as unstable as beach sand beneath your feet.

I remember when I was in elementary school how different kids would tease each other. The kid being teased would often respond by saying, "Sticks and stones may break my bones, but words could never hurt me." Do you remember this? It was cute and believable at the time, but I now understand how wrong that statement was. In fact, sticks and stones could never inflict the level of deep damage that words can and often do. Words are the most powerful and yet the most destructive force in nature. Even scripture tells us that death and life are in the power of the tongue and that we are not to let any corrupt communication come from our mouths (see Proverbs 18:21, Ephesians 4:29).

In Psalms 23:3, King David declares, "He restores my soul." He pens in Psalms 109:22, "For I am poor and needy, and my heart is wounded within me." In order for something to be restored, it first has to have some damage done to it in the first place. This damage we are discussing is damage caused by traumatic emotional events experienced by the person in need of the restoration. The initial trauma in most cases very commonly begins in early childhood and adolescence, and at other times is experienced in early adulthood. Nevertheless, no matter when the emotional trauma was experienced, it is the culprit of an emotional sabotage that has the power and ability to alter the trajectory of emotional wholeness and completeness in a person's life.

When you do a survey of the life of David, you can very easily see that he underwent many battles, attacks on his life, sabotage, rejections, betrayals, accusations, slanders, being misjudged, being misunderstood, and much more. He was even criminalized and was made to run into hiding for doing right and what he was anointed to do when he slayed Goliath. Most of these issues came from people he loved, trusted, befriended, and supported. Imagine for a moment the emotional turmoil that any one of these things would take on you if you were in his shoes today. You can understand some of what he was going through by some of the writings in Psalms, such as Psalms 27 and Psalms 43, for example. These are just two of many such psalms that show some of his inner struggles and plights.

We often think of and hear of David being talked about as a shepherd boy, a warrior, and a king. But do you ever take the time to look into what the weight of those three roles may have cost him emotionally throughout his lifetime? Each of those titles came with the weight and responsibility of expectations from those around him, whether it was family or a friend (and foe when you include those that betrayed him). Sometimes false weights and the unrealistic expectations of others can emotionally bankrupt a person.

As David the young shepherd, he spent a lot of his time separated from others. He had to brave the elements and fight off predators alone in order that the sheep would be fed and protected. Imagine the loneliness and the feelings of isolation, wishing he could be in the comfort of home with his loved ones. In American prisons today, segregation is used as a control measure or a disciplinary tool within the inmate population because most inmates do not want the isolation. As humans, we were created to be social beings, so it is a natural desire to be around others. We find love and security around our loved ones. So, as a shepherd, I can only imagine David's feelings of isolation and feelings of being left out and unloved.

As David the warrior, King Saul, whom David served and was loyal to, turned against him and caused him to become a fugitive, today's equivalent of the FBI's Most Wanted. Numerous times, David put his life on the line while serving Saul, starting with his showdown with Goliath. David's defeat of Goliath led him to Saul's betrayal and to being treated as a criminal. David was labeled as public enemy number one and put on the most wanted list because of Saul's jealousy. Imagine the king putting a hit out on you when all you've done was be loyal. David went from being hailed as a hero to being a fugitive, on the run for the life he sacrificed for the very person he served and respected.

Several times, Saul himself tried to kill David, regardless of David's pleas. Imagine the emotional turmoil and trauma he was going through. David's wife (Saul's daughter) was taken from him by Saul and given to another man while David was out fighting for Saul. Imagine the emotional turmoil and trauma...There was another time where David and his men were away at Ziklag and another enemy—the Amalekites—came in and kidnapped all of their wives and kids and burned their homes to the ground. His own men then threatened to stone him to death. Imagine the emotional turmoil and trauma...David was never a threat to Saul; Saul's own emotions were.

Sometimes it is not the "enemy" that's the problem; it's the "inner-me." Often, the biggest and the baddest enemy that you could ever have is actually the "inner-me."

As if this wasn't enough, fast-forward to later after Saul died and David became king. David's own son Amnon raped his daughter, Tamar (see 2 Samuel 13). Fast-forward from there, David's other son Absalom killed Amnon for this offense and went on the run. Fast-forward from this, this same son Absalom secretly undermined David's leadership, sabotaged his kingship, and took the kingdom from David, and David once again found himself on the run (see 2 Samuel 15 and Psalms 3). Think about the feelings of betrayal. Imagine the emotional trauma and turmoil. As a matter of fact, with the exception of his dealings with Bathsheba, I suggest that most of the issues David had to face were initiated by those close to him. Trying to imagine how David felt during and after all of these issues escapes my imagination at this time.

What I do know is that emotional wounds do not just go away. You cannot just sweep them under the rug. You cannot just ignore them or suppress them. You may have never suffered anything remotely close to the magnitude of anything described in this book so far. But if you have suffered any level of emotional trauma (and most of us have), it is important that you own it and acknowledge it so that you can get the healing you need and deserve.

Emotional trauma can come from a variety of sources, such as rejection as a child, being mishandled as a child (physical abuse, neglect, molestation, rape, verbal abuse, abandonment, being bullied, death of a loved one, etc.). Emotional trauma can come from a variety of sources as adults too, such as divorce or relationship failures, financial hardships, chronic illness, loss of career, etc. No matter the source of the wound or the age you were (are) when the wound occurred, the toxic effects are the same. It may show up and masquerade differently in specific areas of your life, but the sabotaging results are just as damaging.

Let me speak to my guys here for a second. I am especially talking to you right now because I know and understand the challenges of being a man in today's complex and often complicated society. I'm especially speaking to my guys right here because women are more likely to at least attempt to verbalize what they are experiencing emotionally and get it out. We, as men, don't always like to acknowledge our emotions, so we suppress or ignore them (or so we deceptively think). The other option is that we try to group our emotions all together and call it anger, frustration, or "ticked off." No, my brother, you have to correctly identify with what you are really feeling and own it, just like you would describe to a doctor what you are experiencing in your body. Don't allow the pride prison to keep you locked up any longer. Identifying, owning, and expressing your emotions does not make you weak; it can actually strengthen you because you get rid of the weight you inwardly carry. Either you conquer it, or it conquers you—there's no equal cohabitation. You have the power to choose to become proactive, get on the offensive, and overcome, or by default you will become reactive, get on the defensive and are being overcome.

One of the very best things a person can do for themselves in their journey to emotional wholeness and self-care is the free themselves from the expectations of others, and yes, this includes even family members and friends at times. More about this later. Let's get back to David, a Biblical character that I'm sure most of us can identify with.

In each phase of the "roles" that David held as shepherd, warrior, and king, there had to have been tremendous emotional pressures to perform to the expectations of others, even though he was anointed to do so. Sometimes pressures to perform can cause emotional turmoil and physical ailments when not managed properly. Have you or anyone you have known ever been an over-performer? An overachiever? A perfectionist? A controller? Anyone that always has to outdo or out-know everyone else? Been fear driven? Controlled by the residue of past hurts and baggage? Overly guarded? Come on now, be totally honest with yourself—this is your chance for change. If you cannot relate to at least some of this, this book may not be for you. If so, I challenge you to read on.

David is also known for his major downfall with Bathsheba (see 2 Samuel 11). Yet, in spite of this indiscretion, according to scripture, he was considered a man after God's own heart and the apple of His eye. David had an intimacy with God that allowed him to be able to get back into right alignment after his wrong behaviors. There are several instances in scripture where David openly acknowledged the emotional distress and turmoil he was going through. Instead of wallowing in guilt, condemnation, or self-pity, he ran *to* God instead of running *from* Him. Unlike many of us, David owned his emotional state. Often, we would rather deny, mask, or suppress ours and therefore give it a safe haven to simmer beneath the surface and linger for years, even decades.

Isn't it amazing that a person can do 999 things that are good and right, but the one lapse of judgment or mistake they make taints their whole image to others, causing them to misjudge, accuse, gossip, slander, and persecute that person? For some people, they feel better about themselves when they find reasons to judge, condemn, persecute, and criticize others. Why is it that we always want mercy when we mess up, but fail to give mercy to someone else when they need it? This can be a clear indication that there may be some internal issues and the need for some inner healing. Consider the following questions:

> » Have you consistently found yourself working to gain the approval or acceptance of others?

» Do you go out of your way to impress or please others to the point that you neglect and sacrifice your own well-being?

» Do you take criticisms harder than you should?

» Are you overly sensitive to comments from others that may not tickle your fancy or stroke your ego?

» Are you one way with one group of people or in a particular setting and then totally different at home?

» Do you find that you cannot really be yourself with others for fear of not being accepted?

» Are you hiding insecurity and fear by masking it with over-compensation, over-perfectionism, or false machismo?

» Do you find yourself always having to overly explain or overly defend your words, actions, or behaviors?

» Are you overly concerned, or do you worry about how people view you or what they may be thinking of you on a regular basis?

If you can identify with any of the above questions, you may very well be carrying some emotional wounds and are in need of some healing. Even those of you who may have already received some healing, it does not mean there's not a deeper level that's needed. If you cannot readily identify with anything mentioned so far, please consider the possibility that you could have "blind spots" that you are not aware of. Our blind spots are just as the name implies, blind spots in our characters that we don't see because of wounds, filters, pride, and cognitive dissonance. Continue reading and hopefully you will discover where you are by the end of this book.

Chapter 2

COGNITIVE DISSONANCE

Cognitive dissonance occurs when what a person thinks varies significantly from the true reality in a given situation. When a person has not properly healed from traumas and is still carrying residual effects of past damaged emotions, the way they view the world and process information around certain types of situations, scenarios, and events is oftentimes skewed, altered, and tainted by the trauma. The trauma causes them to actually build strongholds and create filters through which any new information passes through. Filters actually restrict how or what the person sees, hears, or experiences within certain types of situations, just like blinds on windows filter out sunlight. When a person has filters, like most of us have had in our own lives, they are totally unaware that their filter even exists. They deny it, justify it, and will fight you to defend it, but remember, they have blinders and cannot see it. Blinders block out and hide our own behaviors to ourselves, and the person is totally unaware of it.

When you attempt to communicate something very clearly to someone that has emotional wounds and filters, what they actually hear is something vastly different from the message that you are trying to convey, and then comes the contention, confusion, and the accusations that follow. What happens is that when they hear certain trigger words, it then activates or triggers a negative, unhealthy emotion that's tied to a negative memory in their subconscious mind from their past that never healed fully, if at all.

So, what happens next is that they quickly transition from trying to understand what is being said to thinking about their own response; their defenses go up, and then the battle begins. When this occurs, the person trying to communicate ends up having to defend or clarify the message they are trying to share with the receiver. The person that's doing the receiving hears attacks, accusations, condemnation, rejection, criticism, and judgment. They're not good enough, not smart enough, or not "whatever" enough. This all happens at the subconscious level within just a millisecond.

This is why I believe that healing has two parts to be complete:

1. actually getting healed, and

2. renewing the mind afterwards to maintain the healing.

For every area where the mind is unrenewed, there is a potential open door that makes you vulnerable and susceptible to "perceived" threats and attacks. This is especially true when dealing with damaged emotions from past soul traumas.

For the sake of making this point more easily relatable, I would like to introduce to you a married couple named Jack and Jill. Jack grew up in a household with several older siblings. As a kid, he always felt like he had to compete with his siblings for his parents' affection, attention, and support. He was the youngest of his siblings, so some activities were not age appropriate for him that his older siblings were able to do, simply due to being several years younger than his closest sibling. Jack often felt left out, not loved, misunderstood, unheard, unseen, mistreated, and as if life was not fair at home. In reality, no good and responsible parent would allow their seven-year-old to engage in some of the activities that they would allow a twelve-year-old to do, would they? In Jack's young mind, his protection actually felt like punishment.

Jill, on the other hand, was the oldest of her siblings. When she was younger, she was the only child in the household for several years until her younger siblings came into the picture. She had been used to receiving all of her parents' and family members' attention, adoration, and affection. For birthdays and holidays, it was "all about Jill"...until the second child was born, and then the third. All of this attention seemingly came to an abrupt halt in her young mind. It felt to her as if all the affections suddenly shifted from being centered on her and placed on her younger sibling...and then another. Like Jack, she often began to feel left out, not loved, misunderstood, unheard, unseen, mistreated, and as if life was not fair at home. At no fault of her own, life had changed from a world where she felt valued and secure to one where she was an afterthought and abandoned, or so it seemed. In all actuality, nothing at all had really changed in regard to her parents' love and affections towards her, but they now had a new baby to care for that required a lot of time and attention. If you are reading this and are a parent, you understand this totally.

The two scenarios above are just two examples out of the countless many that could have been used. Both are very common and create environments that cause emotional wounds that can be and often are carried twenty, thirty, forty, fifty years, or even for a lifetime if not properly dealt with. In both scenarios mentioned above concerning Jack and Jill, the situations they grew up in at home caused them both to develop some major rejection issues, relationship issues, some fears, some negative self-images, and some personal insecurities that followed them into adolescence and on into adulthood relationships.

Now, let's fast-forward. Let's look twenty years down the road when they are married with their own children. The pressures of careers, financial obligations, marriage, parenting, and the weight of a family all piled up on them both. They look so good, happy, and successful on the exterior, but keep in mind that the emotional wounds they sustained as children are still present in their interior foundation but are suppressed, masked, and polished up. In fact, they are not even aware, totally oblivious to the existence of these wounds, even though strong undercurrents hint of them periodically.

A few years down the road, they realize the honeymoon is over. They love each other, but life itself has begun to tear at the seams in them both where there have been unhealed areas that lie beneath the surface. They go through times, like many couples do, where they no longer see eye to eye on some things. They have a fight from time to time, but they never properly resolve them. What they are not realizing is that these unresolved issues are still playing in the background (trauma still speaking) putting a drain on their emotional batteries, just like open apps working in the background on your laptop or smartphone.

Instead of working through their issues, Jill wants to avoid conflict (out of fear) and decides to just keep silent for the sake of keeping the peace (false peace, I might add), so she suppresses toxic thoughts. Jack, on the other hand, wants to talk about it because not doing so makes him keep it inside (suppression leads to depression). Look at the dynamic at hand here—Jill is triggered into silence because she was made to feel bad growing up if she voiced her concerns, so avoiding conflict feels "safe" for her, even though it's not good for her or the relationship. Jack feels like she does not care due to her silence, and this silence triggers the rejection in him because of what he sustained and developed as a child when he felt unheard. In this case, this is where things can go from bad to worse. This scenario can go one of a few different ways.

On another day, they have a disagreement about something very minute and insignificant that got blown way out of proportion. Because of Jack's unhealed childhood emotional wounds and filters, he feels as if Jill is not listening to him and he is unheard, unseen, misunderstood, mistreated, and that life is unfair at home with Jill, and thereby he is unknowingly reliving the wound again within the present-day context of their argument. Jill, on the other hand, because of her unhealed childhood emotional wounds, feels undervalued, not loved, misunderstood, unheard, unseen, and mistreated, and as if life is not fair at home with Jack. She also, in that moment, is reliving the wound from her past. They are both experiencing the "new" situation from that "old" wounded place, and these wounds filter how they are processing the situation.

The residual effects of both Jack and Jill's unhealed emotional trauma that began decades earlier created an element of dysfunction embedded within each of them. This dysfunction has silently stalked and followed them into their marriage. Because of the pressures of life, it is now getting triggered, causing them to turn on each other and treat one another as the enemy when, realistically speaking, the "inner-me" is the real enemy here. They are like unsuspecting puppets being controlled by an indiscernible internal puppet master. They both are processing the minute and insignificant issue through a very serious emotional filter that is blocking truth from them both and keeping them in the dark about themselves and each other. Does any of this seem familiar at all to you?

Chapter 3

FILTERS

Filters were briefly mentioned in the previous section, so let's unpack and discuss these filters in quite a bit more detail next. We will discuss Jack and Jill more as well. Normally, the various types of filters we use every day work for us and not against us. They are simple in how they work and are designed to protect our assets from becoming liabilities. Most of the time, they are relatively inexpensive in comparison to the damage they prevent. It's cheap insurance for preventing potentially expensive problems, failures, and repairs. For example, a water filter filters out toxic debris and contaminants that can cause damage to your health. Air filters keep the air in our homes clean and safe to breathe and they also protect us from excess dust, toxic pollutants, and allergens. A car oil filter works by filtering out filth and debris that is contained in the oil that could get into the engine and cause catastrophic failure. To put it into perspective, a $20 oil filter can protect a $100,000 car from engine failure.

Filters caused by emotional traumas and wounds are very real, and actually alter the way we think, feel, process, and experience the world around us. These types of filters are a horse of a different color altogether and cause catastrophic effects by working against us and not for us. These filters are not cheap but are extremely costly to us in various areas of our lives. Whenever a person experiences an emotional trauma, from the onset of that trauma forward, they process life through the lens of that wound(s) until they are fully healed, if ever. In actuality, the information they see and hear is skewed as it is processed through their damaged emotions. They build strongholds and apply filters on the false foundation of that wound, and the effects just compile as more and more weights and wounds are added on. These filters are major liabilities and have the potential to cause catastrophic failures in relationships, careers, emotional wellbeing, physical health, and in any area of a person's life. We build strongholds in our minds for certain scenarios so that we can self-protect from what we may feel is harmful to us.

Filters can blind us to our own negative behaviors while causing us to skew and magnify the behaviors we see in others. Truthfully speaking, sometimes the thing you're fighting about has nothing at all to do with the one you are fighting with. Certain actions or words activate them into a fight-or-flight response because they are sensing a threat subconsciously. To be honest, the person with the filter doesn't even really hear or see accurately once they are triggered because their reasoning is now based on skewed information they have processed, and they are reacting from a place of damaged emotions. This damage has caused their logic to become distorted, and strong filters with negative beliefs attached to them are now in full swing. When you add the trauma, the triggers, the filters, and the distortions together and create a situation where strong emotions are active, this is a recipe for potential disaster in communication.

It is very common for damaged emotions and filters to trigger a person into becoming hyper-sensitive to threats, or should I say "perceived" threats, because most of the time the threat is only an imagined one. This is prime evidence of past unhealed trauma still speaking in that person's life. Think of the Jack and Jill scenario regarding cognitive dissonance. The exact same thing applies when it comes to filters as well. In the scenario, both Jack and Jill had cognitive dissonance and there were filters operating in them that caused it.

We commonly call this trauma "baggage" but it's much more than that. Think about baggage in the following example. If you have ever flown on a plane, you know that the airlines charge additional fees above the ticket prices for your extra baggage that is over the set normal limit of how much can be brought onboard. Additional fees are charged because this extra baggage is taking up limited space, and more importantly, it adds extra weight to the plane. Keep in mind that each plane has a weight limit, so there is a preset estimated amount of fuel that should be used for each flight that's based on distance, altitude, speed, and the weight of the plane. Any weight added from extra baggage causes the planes to burn more fuel, costing the airlines more, and this takes away from their profits. In other words, it's costing the airline valuable profits whenever passengers travel with extra baggage.

I have a few questions I would like you to think about:

» What is your emotional baggage costing you?

» How much is it really weighing you down?

» How much of your fuel and energy is being drained because of it?

» How much is it stifling your potential and stagnating your life's purpose? Is it harmful to your relationships? To your emotional health? To your physical health and body?

If you do not believe that carrying unhealed emotional wounds is costing you, think again. I submit to you that if you do have unhealed damaged emotions, it is costing you and it may have potentially already costed you more than you even realize. My sincere hope is that you will recognize just how much so before you get to the end of this book series and that you can recover all that was lost or has been stolen from you.

These filters can wreak havoc on communications and damage relationships by creating a lot of confusion, contention, and toxicity. As I previously stated, when a negative emotion or negative subconscious memory gets activated (triggered) in a person, they then stop listening to understand what is being said and they immediately begin processing a defensive response to what they thought they heard. Again, this is a perceived threat, not an actual one, but it is real to them because of trauma, damaged emotions, cognitive dissonance, filters, and triggers.

Filters have a very real way of twisting, distorting, and even disrupting effective communications, causing them to sometimes become confusing and toxic. The negative impact of filters is in direct proportion to the level of healing that is needed. This has been the cause of so many miscommunications, misunderstandings, accusations, offenses, arguments, altercations, fights, rivalries, even divorces. A clear indicator of this is when you react to situations based on your feelings rather than based on truth, sound reasoning, facts, or clear logic.

The person who is impacted by these filters can become very rigid in their stance and beliefs in a particular situation, inflexible and unable to receive anything that contradicts whatever they already believe. We will dive into more detail on what drives this type of thinking in part two of this book. Remember this truth: Feelings Are NOT Facts. Trust me, we have all been there, whether we were the sender or the receiver of the communication. I'm sure as you are reading this, you can think of some scenarios where you can look back and see this in action. It is a very powerfully destructive and disruptive issue, so the more you can understand it, the more equipped you will be to overcome it within your own lives and your relationships with others.

The most difficult thing about filters is that the person who has them is mostly oblivious to recognizing them and will deny them. Plus, they often resist conversations that could help set them free and can become defensive at the mention of their filters. Keep in mind that it is likely this started in childhood, adolescence, or early adulthood and is possibly deeply embedded within their foundations and subconscious minds. So it is a very sensitive issue from the start. If this is you, the reader, I believe it is time for your healing. In fact, I believe that it is important for you to get healed before trying to help anyone else get healed. If not, you could open yourself up for more triggers to being activated and it would cause more harm than good if you were to experience any type of emotional setbacks.

If you want to overcome your emotional wounds and conquer the negative consequences they are causing in your life, you cannot just treat the symptoms. The symptoms are specifically the negative unhealthy emotions and the adverse behaviors or reactions tied to them. You have to get to the root cause or the foundation of the emotional wounds, which in most cases, you have to discover its actual origins. The foundation of it all is actually the trauma itself and the thoughts that are being produced because of it. The emotional wounds, the filters, the cognitive dissonance, the triggers are all working together to wreak havoc on your peace, your relationships with others (as well as with yourself), your potential, your dreams, your health (physical and emotional), your children, and just about every area in life you can think of.

Just to be clear, your educational status, career or financial success, titles, or heightened social status does not mean you are exempt. I may mention this several times before the end of this book, but you have to understand the importance of the next statement I am going to make: *Thoughts create emotions. Emotions drive behaviors. Behaviors produce thoughts and emotions.* Understanding this simple but true concept will be a vital step towards your healing journey.

Whenever you are feeling certain feelings, it is directly tied to you thinking certain thoughts.

Here is a very simple but effective practical application exercise that you can start doing today: The very next time you are feeling a little disturbed, heavy, depressed, anxious, angry, frustrated, or any negative emotion, trace back to when you started feeling this. Most of the time, you should be able to identify some thought patterns that you were having just before you started experiencing the negative emotions. Or maybe you can think of a recent time you were experiencing some negative emotions. Think back and take a panoramic view of the scenario with this new lens. Trace back to what you experienced just before the emotions were triggered. You may have moved on from whatever happened in your conscious mind because you had to work, live, or because of other responsibilities. The problem was that it was still operating in the background in your subconscious mind, speaking to you in ways that you may have been unaware of or chose to ignore. You may have moved on from "it," but did it really move on from you? Let me make this disclaimer: this is not the case if you have a medical condition or side effects from medications that cause these emotions, but I will say that negative unhealthy thoughts and emotions can create and cause medical conditions to manifest in your body.

Understanding these things is a dangerously vital lifeline in ministry and faith-based organizations. I use the term "dangerously" here because, from leadership to laymen, we collectively have the potential to contaminate tens of thousands of other people who follow us or that we are connected to. For this reason, I appeal to you leaders (and non-leaders) that serve in any capacity in any type of organization (school, ministry, business, etc.) because we often are imprisoned by the titles and responsibilities that go along with them. I submit to you that healing is for you also. If you serve the people as a leader, it is okay to take at least a mini sabbatical from time to time so that you can receive back that which you have constantly poured out to others. You cannot pour from an empty or contaminated vessel. As a matter of fact, I have taken several myself. It does not always have to be a long break; sometimes just a few days or couple of weeks can work wonders in helping you to unplug and reset. This goes for caregivers as well, and anyone that has to shoulder the responsibility of carrying the weight of others. Your self-care is very important and much needed. No one is exempt. No one...even Jesus rested.

Chapter 4

THINKING CYCLES

Understand this and it will absolutely revolutionize your life: Thoughts create emotions. Emotions drive behaviors. Behaviors produce thoughts and emotions. If you want to change behavior and just go after the behavior itself, you will fail. If you want to change an emotion and go after just that emotion itself, you will fail in this also. Yes, you may possibly experience some short-term relief, but it will not be a permanent or consistent change, just a temporary one because it will still be based on a feeling. If you want to change either emotions or behaviors, you must go after the thoughts (the root) that create the emotion that drives the behavior...period. In the root you will find the problem, and in the root, you will find the solution. The negative emotions and the negative behaviors associated with them are just symptoms of the negative thoughts that created them in the first place. You see, it all ties back to the thoughts of the mind. This is why we are instructed in Romans 12:2 that we are not to give in to the pressures and influences of this world, but instead to renew our minds.

In the fire triangle, there needs to be three things for a fire to burn: a heat source, oxygen, and fuel. If you remove any of the elements in the fire triangle, especially the fuel, then the fire cannot burn. Likewise, when it comes to the triangle of your thoughts, emotions, and behaviors, you have to remove the thoughts (the actual fuel) so that you can change the emotions, actions or behaviors associated with them permanently. The thoughts are doing the driving, and whatever follows is always a result of them.

As a matter of fact, when a child goes through emotionally traumatic experiences and suffers wounded emotions as a result, their emotional development in that area from that point forward can be stagnated. Years later as an adult, if they are triggered by a highly emotional event, they very easily overreact to it. This can be something seemingly small or insignificant, and they often will demonstrate behavior that's way out of normal character in relation to what it should be. So, in essence, it's the child version or the six-year-old version of themselves manifesting the behaviors in their now adult life even at forty, fifty, sixty, or seventy plus years old. This is what is called "arrested development." Their emotional development was "arrested" or frozen in the area where the trauma was experienced, and they have been stuck there ever since. Sure, they were able to develop normally in many other areas, but that one area is still taboo and is easily triggered.

Many of us live in this space and attribute it to "this is just how I am" or as normal. In a case such as this, the emotional development was damaged, stunted, halted, delayed, hindered, altered, etc. This is exactly the place where many of us are today as adults. So we carry this residue over into adulthood, make adult decisions, enter adult relationships, careers, ministries, and parenthood with this arrested development and end up recycling the dysfunctions that come with it, even into the next generation.

Many people have been mentally imprisoned by certain patterns of thinking due to their unhealed, damaged emotions. More than likely, these people will experience repeated cycles of negative and toxic behaviors when triggered within certain types of situations. These include pain, despair, disappointment, depression, control, offensiveness, defensiveness, dysfunctional behaviors, insecurities, hypersensitivity, over-reactiveness, fears, anxieties, anger, frustrations, etc. There's a whole host of other very common expressions and indicators of internal traumas that are "speaking" in their lives, but they don't realize it. Yes, trauma does speak in various ways, but there are way too many to mention here.

By now, though, I'm sure you are starting to get the picture. When wounded emotions are operating behind people's decisions, actions, belief systems, and behaviors, it creates cyclical mindsets and strongholds that are not always easily recognizable because they are often masked by over-compensating behaviors. They typically justify their beliefs and actions that mindset produces because they feel that it's normal and "safe," but in reality, they are just in survival or self-protect mode and don't realize it. It is also common for them to have a victim mentality and never seem to take accountability or be responsible for their actions. One reason is that their filters, blinders, and cognitive dissonance will very often block them from seeing themselves as in the wrong. Pride is very instrumental in this also because of the blind spots it creates, but this is a whole different topic for a different day.

Next to receiving emotional healing, renewing the mind, according to Romans 12:2, is very instrumental and is one of the most important things a person can ever do for themselves. With healing and deliverance, you can be set free, but without renewing your mind as part of that process there's no way to remain free, so there's a two-step process that has to take place to guarantee your long-lived success. You cannot solve problems with the same mindset you had when they were created in the first place. Who the Son sets free is free indeed (and in deed). Without being armed with a refreshed, revived, restored, and renewed mind, you will continue to have blind spots, filters, strongholds, triggers, dysfunctions, and emotional bondage, no matter how long you've been in church, no matter your title, your calling, your anointing, your gifts, your knowledge of scripture, your education, your career, your accolades, your accomplishments, or how old you are.

We sometimes develop strongholds in our minds in an effort to protect ourselves from harm or anything that poses a threat to our well-being, and sadly carry them for decades, unknowingly. Strongholds don't just dissolve themselves. Emotional wounds do not just heal themselves. These wounds have to be acknowledged that they are even there and very purposefully worked through. Emotional wounds can never be healed by suppressing them or denying their existence. You will never conquer what you don't first confront, and whatever you do not conquer conquers you. These wounds have to be uncovered and understood so their power can be broken. You have to understand how they work and what that looks like. Further, you have to understand and be able to identify their origins. Then the negative effects of the trauma can be strategically neutralized, and all traces, residue, and baggage removed from your life completely.

Just imagine for a moment that you can experience life with no more baggage. No more triggers. No more filters. No more blind spots. No more fears, anxieties, anger, or dysfunctions being recycled from generation to generation. Most of the people that I've known to be set free and healed never realized how weighted down they were until after they experienced true freedom. What you do not have power over may just have power over you.

When a truck is pulling a heavy load; it will consume more fuel than it would without the load behind it. Even a large ship sits lower in the water and consumes more fuel when laden with hundreds of tons of cargo. My question to you today is what is your baggage costing you? How much of your energy is being consumed because of the excess weight of emotional baggage and wrong mindsets every day? How much of your potential is being stifled because of excess baggage? The crazy thing about baggage is, the longer you carry it, the more used to it you get and after a while you forget that it is even on your shoulder. It becomes your "new normal" and you just forget it's even there.

Here's a scary thought: whatever emotional baggage from past trauma you carry as a parent gets recycled into your children's lives. Yes, they may inherit your DNA, and they may have several of your traits, look just like you, and have some of your tendencies, too. Yet, the problem is, we recycle our mindsets also. We have a tendency to become the very things we hate, and in our efforts to be good parents and to give them the very best of what we did not have as kids, we inadvertently pass on some of those wrong thought processes and dysfunctions as well. This is especially real if you carried trauma and damaged emotions before becoming a parent.

Truthfully, we may never even realize the extent of what has been passed down until they are older, and we begin to wonder why they do what they do or why they act like they act, seemingly without reason or logic. You may even think to yourself or say out loud, "You weren't raised like that." And you may be right, they may not have been raised *like* that, but could it be that they were raised *in* that? This does not mean you were not a good parent. That just means you are human and did the very best you knew to do at the time because of what you yourself may have inherited. In my humble opinion, I believe that every adult should go through at least a basic level of healing and deliverance before entering into marriage, parenthood, ministry, or careers. I know this is wishful thinking, but just imagine if it were possible. Think of the difference it would have made in your own decisions and how your life may have been different.

Many of our biggest miscalculations, mistakes, and misjudgments have been made based on filters, blinders, temporary emotions, or skewed logic based on erroneous thinking of some type. Trace some of your biggest disappointments back and you will see that there were some filters or errors in your thinking somewhere down the line. To all my brothers and sisters, I submit to you today that these cycles never stop on their own. Seasons change, but cycles just keep repeating themselves, regenerating themselves with no end until something drastic changes. Be the cycle breaker in your family, in your community, and in your circle of influence. By doing so, you can change the lives of many today and of future generations. If you can just change the life of one, let it at least be yours. In order to break these cycles, you have to go after the mindset that created them in the first place. You see, it all comes back to how we are thinking and processing information.

Again, I have stated this before, and it's worth repeating here: thoughts create emotions. Emotions drive behaviors. Behaviors influence thoughts and emotions. You are feeling like you are feeling and doing what you are doing because you are thinking like you are thinking. Most often we focus on how we are actually feeling from day-to-day at any given moment, but when was the last time you actually thought about what you were thinking about?

Think about this: remember the last time you were really upset with someone about something they did or did not do, or something they said? I'm willing to bet the more you thought about the incident, the worse you ended up feeling about it. When you continue to repeat the offense in your mind over and over and over, this is called "ruminating." When you continue to replay a scenario over and over in your memory or ruminate, you produce more and more negative emotions about it. You stack up or build layers of negative emotions until you end up having a very negative reaction to whatever the situation is. When this happens, you have actually just "thought" yourself into depression, frustration, anger, regret, resentment, bitterness, fear, rejection, offensiveness, defensiveness, etc. Yes, YOU did it. When you recycle negative thoughts, it will positively rob you of your peace, your joy, and your energy. Regardless of what the issue is, it was YOUR thoughts that put you in the mood you ended up in.

You have to understand, offense is *taken*. No one has the power to offend us unless we give power away by *taking* (accepting) the offense, and this is based on how you decide to process what's been presented. I am in no way over-simplifying it or saying it's easy, but just like we choose to take offense, we can actually choose to not take offense. Thanks be to God for giving us the power of choice and the freedom to do so!

We get offended because of the "meaning" that we ourselves attach to situations and incidents. This is done so quickly and at such a subconscious level that we have no idea it's even happening, and all we are left to know is how we are feeling as a result. We never understand how we even got there, so we blame and punish the other person for how we feel. In essence, we give them the power over our feelings, whether it be to make us upset or to make us happy, when the truth of the matter is that you are responsible for your own emotional well-being—no one else is. Men that are reading this, take your power back. Women that are reading this, take your power back.

If you really think about it and dissect it, there is often just a very brief instant of processing before we give a negative reaction to a comment or a situation where we actually decide which way we will react. This all happens within a split second, so you have to be very aware of it and it takes practice. Many of us were not taught to be self-aware, so in certain instances, we instead are on autopilot and our reactions are automatic. Practice mentally slowing things down and not giving a reaction to negative situations or comments. That's right, your very first reaction should be no reaction at all. First, you should actually pause, slow things down in your mind, then process it and analyze it from a neutral place of peace rather than just reacting to a negative stimulation. Secure your inner peace before responding or reacting and then you won't have to fight to restore what you already have...your peace. Remember this, the feelings you are experiencing are not the problem, they are just a symptom of the negative thoughts that are actively creating, recycling, and feeding the negative feelings. Please take a few moments to reread this paragraph again and let it sink in.

Let's take a look at the prophet Elijah for a moment in 1 Kings 18 and 19. Elijah was a man who followed God and performed mighty miracles throughout the land. In fact, one of his greatest miracles occurred just before his greatest mishap. On one hand was one of the biggest showdowns in recorded Biblical history between the prophets of Baal and Asherah and the God who answers by fire (see 1 Kings 18:20–40). On the other hand was one of the biggest mysteries in recorded Biblical history: how a man walking in such incredible miraculous power could have this huge emotional reaction in such a big way to a single threat from Jezebel that it caused him to potentially alter the rest of his life and ministry (1 Kings 19:1–4). Her single threat triggered such a fear and a fight-or-flight response in Elijah that had previously not been seen in his life, or in anyone in Scripture up to that point. How can such boldness and miracle-working power be demonstrated, and yet such staggering life-paralyzing fear operate in the same person like this? This was always a total mystery to me until I learned about emotional wounds, filters, triggers, ANTs (Automatic Negative Thoughts, will be discussed in the next section), and emotional responses.[1]

The Bible states that Elijah "saw" the threats made to him by Jezebel (see verse 3), and he rose and ran for his life. In essence, what this means is that Elijah actually imagined (thought) her threats were coming true, he became fearful (emotion), and then this fear caused him to run away (behavior). Remember, thoughts create emotions, and emotions drive behaviors. It was Elijah's thoughts and the imagery of her threats that produced the fear response. Power demonstrated one moment; paralyzing fear demonstrated the next.

How many more recorded miracles did Elijah perform after this? How much more of his purpose was fulfilled after this? What was it in Elijah's life or background that caused such a response, which shortened his ministry? If you read further, you will clearly see in verse 16 that God directed him to anoint Elisha in his place. In other words, Elijah was done for. Whatever it was that he imagined happening to him from Jezebel stifled him. How can such a powerful person who had just defeated several hundred prophets of Baal and Asherah react in such a way because of a single person? What was broken in Elijah?

You see, even our gifts and anointings cannot outrun the traumatic effects of damaged emotions, strongholds, filters, blinders, triggers, and wrong mindsets. The Bible is not clear about what may have happened in Elijah's life, and I dare not speculate. All I am saying is, hmmm...something was definitely wrong in that scenario and there is a great deal to learn from it.

Chapter 5

--------•--------

ANTs (Automatic Negative Thoughts)

*"For from within, out of the heart of men, proceed evil thoughts,
adulteries, fornications, murders, thefts, covetousness, wickedness,
deceit, lasciviousness, an evil eye, blasphemy, pride, foolishness"*

Mark 7:21–22

When you really pay attention to this scripture, you observe
that the foundation of all the evil things mentioned is the "evil
thoughts." Then, everything else that follows is a result of these evil
thoughts. In other words, the thoughts are the origin, root cause,
or point of entry for everything in that scripture. The foundation
is the most important part of any building or structure because
everything else is built on that foundation. If the foundation is
not built correctly, it will not be strong enough to bear the weight
of that structure. As a result, the entire structure, everything
that's built upon it, and everyone in it could be at risk. With
this being said, it is of the most importance that the structure's
foundation is built according to the blueprint. It is also of the
utmost importance that the blueprint is designed correctly. This
is true for any type of building, no matter how large or small.

As a people, thoughts are the foundation of our lives. As a matter of fact, regardless of how strong you are in your faith, no matter how strong you are in your gifts, no matter how prominent you are in your walk, your thought life can veto, override, overrule, and overthrow your destiny and life's purpose. One thing I have come to understand as it pertains to people is that no one or nothing can push past a person's intellect or mindset. This is especially true when wounded emotions are operating.

Have you ever had a negative experience with someone and then sometime down the road you see that person or hear their name mentioned and have negative thoughts or feelings about them? Most of the time this happens without us even realizing it. It could be months or even years since the offense occurred, and yet the very sight or sound of that person's name triggers a negative response in you. I believe that some of you reading this are bearing witness to this right now.

Have you ever experienced when a close family member or particular person makes a certain type of comment concerning you that you get triggered into negative thoughts and emotions without you even thinking about it or realizing it? Do you automatically respond with a negative remark or comment when you feel like you're being accused or attacked by them? If any of this describes you, you have ANTs (Automatic Negative Thoughts). These ANTs are automatic, uninvited, undetected, unwelcomed, and undesirable. ANTs are negative thoughts that just automatically pop up in your mind without warning.

This automatically occurs due to the fact that those thoughts have been embedded in your mind because of an offense you have suffered. Please understand that when this happens, it could actually be your old wound talking to you in an undiscerning way. Sometimes this wound may just be to your pride or ego, other times it may be legitimate damage to the soul. (Note: a big ego is a sign of over-compensating for insecurity, by the way.) Either way, you have ANTs and you need to get rid of them!

I grew up in the south and loved to spend time doing outdoor activities. I remember as a boy, my friends and I would sometimes play with bugs, such as ants. Today, I no longer play with bugs of any type, so whenever I see a bug inside, I get rid of it right away. This is especially true when it comes to ants. If you ever see ants inside of your house, get rid of them as quickly as you possibly can, or you will end up with dozens of them before long. But the problem starts with only just a single ant.

When an ant locates a food source, it communicates to the other ants and leaves a scent trail for the others in the colony to follow to that food source. This is why you see ants orderly following the same trail back and forth from the colony to the food. Even the Bible talks about the diligence of ants in Proverbs 6:6–8. Ants always work together, systematically and inter-dependently. Ants are some of the strongest insects ever created because a single ant can carry fifty times its own body weight. They also fight viciously to protect and defend their colonies. They are a real nuisance if they come into your home because they can come through the tiniest of openings, and it's challenging to keep them out once they locate a reliable food source.

Are you wondering why in the world I am talking about ants and what do ants have to do with emotional healing? I'm glad you asked. The same way ants work together, and are very strong and well organized, your ANTs do the same. ANTs and negative beliefs work interdependently and they strengthen and reinforce one another. One of the ways that ANTs are most destructive in relationships is that they distort facts the same way filters distort facts. ANTs can also be small projections or glimpses of your overall limiting belief system and are often built on thinking errors. (Thinking errors will be discussed in part two of this book.)

ANTs are not always easily detectable because they are automatic and can be challenging to overcome if you're not aware that they exist. Most of the time, we are not even aware, so we just follow along with whatever our past traumas silently dictate to us to think. So with this being said, self-awareness or mind-awareness is your very best weapon of defense against them. Your chance for successfully defeating your ANTs grows tremendously once you are alerted to their presence and understand how they are working within you.

Please understand also that ANTs are evidence of triggers. Being able to identify your own ANTs and how they are working against you will give you the ability to understand how your beliefs (thinking) lead you into those specific emotions and behaviors that you experience. Unhealthy thinking leads to unhealthy emotions, which leads to unhealthy behaviors, which leads to unhealthy thinking, which leads to unhealthy emotions, which leads to unhealthy behaviors...and the cycle continues until it is broken. To get the desired change, you must interrupt the patterns and break cycles that drive you.

One of the most effective ways of dealing with your ANTs is to first understand what your triggers and trigger situations are. Once you are able to identify your triggers, you should be able to connect the dots from your triggers to your ANTs. These triggers are unhealed areas, and they are sabotaging your life. These triggers are what's been activating you into some of those negative emotions and behavior patterns. Most of the time, it happens so quickly you don't even have time to think about it, nor do you realize what's happening until after it has happened.

Triggers can cause us to think in extreme ways, and in turn, to react in extreme ways, because our thinking is driving the feeling, which is driving the behaving. Usually, whenever a person is thinking, feeling, and behaving in extreme ways, it is difficult to get through to them because they don't leave much room for adjustments or corrections in their thinking. When this is the case, the person is very likely subjective to whatever they already believe and can often become resistant until the feelings subside. If this describes you, you have become victimized by your own mindset, and you have become a prisoner of your past trauma. Being more objective and flexible is a much healthier approach and can yield much better results in your life.

Let me say this, your very own thoughts can lie to you and create all types of unnecessary negative unhealthy emotions and toxic behaviors, stress, drama, and confusion in your relationships. They can very easily hijack your life in some destructive and disruptive ways. I love how Second Corinthians 10:4–5 describes how we should be casting down arguments and bringing thoughts into captivity. It's telling us how to be free if we would just do what it says. These "arguments" are the reasonings in our thoughts that go against truth and bring us into bondage. If we don't take our thoughts captive, they can take us captive. What we should do is bring our thoughts under a spotlight and evaluate them for truth before accepting them because they could be based on untruths or half-truths, which are still lies. In other words, arrest your thoughts and inspect them to see if you can trust allowing them to produce emotions in you before giving them the wheel in situations that can have the tendency to turn volatile or highly emotional. Are your thoughts based on facts or just feelings? Remember, feelings are not facts and can change directions at any moment like the wind, but facts will remain no matter what. Feelings can be driven by situations or circumstances, but facts remain constant. You can't always trust feelings (could be distorted by toxic thoughts), but you can always trust facts that are built on real truth.

Take a moment to read Genesis 3:1–6. Pay particular attention to verse 6 when it says, "So when the woman *saw* that the tree was good for good, that it was pleasant to the eyes, and a tree desirable to make one wise" (emphasis mine). Eve saw (imagined) that the tree was good for food based on the deception the enemy presented to her. She was manipulated by the enemy's projected lies, and he used her own imagination against her. This triggered her to imagine (see) something that was based on trickery and deception.

What mechanism was operating in Eve that caused her to allow herself to be deceived and triggered in the first place? I doubt seriously that it was an emotional wound or some type of trauma. What was it then? Was there an element of pride that opened that door? Was it fear of losing something she already had or did not need?

What you have to realize is that sometimes pride can actually be rooted in fear. The Bible tells us in 2 Timothy 1:7 that God has not given us a spirit of fear, but of love, of power, and of a sound mind. Also, 1 John 4:18 informs us that fear involves torment. So, in essence, when pride is in operation, that person sometimes reacts to situations based on a hidden insecurity, fear of losing something, or based on the illusion that they are in control in the first place. What has pride deceived or triggered you into imagining? We have been instructed to cast down imaginations (2 Corinthians 10:5), and when we don't, we often sabotage our own selves but blame others for this.

Chapter 6

---·---

NOW THE WORK BEGINS

Let us pray:

Heavenly Father, I pray for those reading this book and searching for that inner-healing and emotional wholeness that they are in need of. I stand in agreement that who the Son sets free is free indeed and where the Spirit of the Lord is, there's liberty. I pray for them to have supernatural strength and might to stand, the boldness of a lion to conquer their fears, and the supernatural peace of God that passes all understanding to persevere through their process. I decree over them the releasing of healing virtue and power and that all their chains, yokes, shackles, and emotional bondages will be totally destroyed. I pray strength to their faith and resolve, for we know that without faith, it is impossible to please You. I stand with them in agreement with Your Word that healing is the children's bread, and no good thing will You withhold from them. I pray for total restoration in their lives. Let healing rain, let healing reign. We thank you and seal this prayer in Jesus Christ's mighty name. Amen.

The workbook exercises in this book are designed to be tools that will bring you into a place of self-awareness by helping you to uncover and confront those old emotional wounds so they can be removed from your life. Please be intentional and make the time that's needed to put forth the necessary effort so you can finally get the healing that

God has for you. Hurts are part of life, but they don't have to define or alter your life. I encourage you to pray and ask God to show you the areas where healing is needed and then commit yourself to the process that will begin your healing journey. The long-term rewards will far outweigh any of the short-term discomforts that may be part of your process. Remember, freedom is priceless, but not costless. You deserve it and it's yours for the taking today. You can never overcome what you will not first own. If you do not confront it, you will not conquer it. If you refuse to own it, then by default it owns you.

I suggest that you reread the chapters. Let's begin:

1. Based on what you have read thus far, name the signs that you see within yourself that indicate you may need some emotional healing. What behaviors do you display when you are upset when others do not do what you want them to do? These will be clear indicators and clues that healing is needed. Be as specific and detailed as possible:

_____

_____

_____

_____

_____

_____

_____

_____

_____

_____

_____

_____

_____

_____

2. Based on what you read in Chapter 1, list the emotional traumas that you recognize and can identify within yourself. To be most effective, you may have to go back into your childhood years. This is where most emotional trauma begins. Do not be in a rush to get past this section. Take some time to unpack this. This is where you have to actually label your emotions. Using terms like "upset" or "mad" is too general and will not be specific enough. Naming them will help you to identify them properly and will help with self-awareness as you go through the exercises.

_____

_____

_____

_____

_____

_____

_____

_____

_____

_____

_____

_____

_____

_____

3. As discussed in Chapter 2, note the instances that you can recognize and identify areas where you have cognitive dissonance operating in your life. You may have to refer back to this task periodically and add to the list as you become more self-aware and as your understanding is increased. You can ask those closest to you for some examples of when they tried conveying something to you, but you heard something different. Think of yourself in the Jack and Jill scenario. Can you see any of the tendencies mentioned within yourself?

_____

_____

_____

_____

_____

_____

_____

_____

_____

_____

_____

_____

4. Throughout each day, make quick notes of your true feelings and emotions while you are in the process of going through the exercises. A lot of thoughts and emotions that have been buried can resurface during this time, so it's important to acknowledge them by noting them. For example, anger, sadness, guilt, resentment, unforgiveness, bitterness, hatred, jealousy, envy, regret, etc. Think about all the different ingredients that go into your favorite dish. Individually, they may be good, but not as good as they are collectively, right? For this exercise, the thoughts, emotions, and behaviors are all individual ingredients that produce the version of "YOU" that you live out every day.

_____

_____

_____

_____

_____

_____

_____

_____

_____

_____

_____

5. How much damage have you really suffered?

_____

_____

_____

_____

_____

_____

_____

_____

_____

_____

_____

_____

_____

_____

_____

_____

_____

_____

6. Identify your thinking cycles, as discussed in Chapter 4.

_____

_____

_____

_____

_____

_____

_____

_____

_____

_____

_____

_____

_____

_____

_____

_____

_____

_____

_____

7. Where did you learn to think in these ways?

_____

_____

_____

_____

_____

_____

_____

_____

_____

_____

_____

_____

_____

_____

_____

_____

8. In what ways can you change your thinking patterns in order to change your behaviors?

_____

_____

_____

_____

_____

_____

_____

_____

_____

_____

_____

_____

_____

_____

_____

9. What situation(s) really broke you?

_____

_____

_____

_____

_____

_____

_____

_____

_____

_____

_____

_____

_____

_____

_____

_____

_____

10. How much damage have you really suffered?

_____

_____

_____

_____

_____

_____

_____

_____

_____

_____

_____

_____

_____

_____

_____

_____

_____

_____

11. How have you typically dealt with the issue at hand?

_____

_____

_____

_____

_____

_____

_____

_____

_____

_____

_____

_____

_____

_____

_____

_____

_____

_____

12. How does your family normally deal with these issues?

_____

_____

_____

_____

_____

_____

_____

_____

_____

_____

_____

_____

_____

_____

_____

_____

_____

_____

13. How much healing have you really received?

_____

_____

_____

_____

_____

_____

_____

_____

_____

_____

_____

_____

_____

_____

_____

_____

_____

14. How much recycling of these issues has your family produced?

_____

_____

_____

_____

_____

_____

_____

_____

_____

_____

_____

_____

_____

_____

_____

_____

15. How much healing have they received?

_____

_____

_____

_____

_____

_____

_____

_____

_____

_____

_____

_____

_____

_____

_____

_____

_____

16. Do your ABCs:

Each day/night, designate some time to write down the details about the exercises above. Include the thoughts, emotions, and behaviors that are being produced as a result of the exercises. This is an important step in the process of your healing and should not be taken lightly. Whatever thoughts and emotions that you have suppressed may come up during this time. It is important that you allow them to do so. You do have to deny or suppress them any longer. As you are journaling, be intentional, be specific, and most importantly, be consistent. Start by taking a moment to trace your day back to any events that may have had any negative impact on you. Once you do this, follow the steps below.

A. Activating event

» What was the event(s) that activated or triggered any negative thoughts or emotions in you throughout the day?

_____

_____

_____

_____

_____

_____

_____

_____

_____

_____

_____

_____

_____

_____

_____

_____

B. Behavior

» What was your first initial thought (what you really wanted to do)?

_____

_____

_____

_____

_____

_____

_____

» What behavior did you actually demonstrate as a reaction to the event mentioned above?

_____

_____

_____

_____

_____

_____

_____

C. Consequence

» What was the consequence(s) of your behavior?

_____

_____

_____

_____

_____

_____

_____

» Did it produce more negative thoughts, feelings, or behaviors?

_____

_____

_____

_____

_____

_____

_____

» Did you leave you with any regret, remorse, or satisfaction?

_____

_____

_____

_____

_____

_____

_____

» What steps can you take to prevent repeating any negative consequences in the future?

_____

_____

_____

_____

_____

_____

_____

To bring balance, you can also use the ABCs steps to track your positive thoughts, behaviors, and to show your progress and your growth.

By now, I am hopeful and optimistic that you are beginning to see how everything that's been discussed all ties together to bring you to the place where you have been for so long. Now, by knowing this, you can be much more effective in navigating and overcoming everyday situations that life can bring. In conclusion, this book is designed to get you started on your journey towards healing and restoration into wholeness. Though it can and should yield some very positive results in your life, it by no means covers every possible scenario or situation. It is not designed to take the place of any professional help if you need it. It is designed to be another tool that you can actually apply on a daily basis. But, just like any other type of tool, they only work if you use them properly. Stay tuned for part two of this book, where we will dive deeper into how to identify some very common thinking errors that often sabotage and hijack the trajectory of our lives and families each and every day in every way.

Endnotes

1. Dana, Jamie. 2018. "How to Stomp out ANTs: Automatic Negative Thoughts." Elevate Counseling. February 2, 2018. https://elevatecounselingaz.com/ants-automatic-negative-thoughts/#:~:text=Ants%20are%20a%20fitting%20metaphor.

For bookings or more information visit:
Dominion-LYFE.org

or send email to:
Stevenallen@dominion-lyfe.org